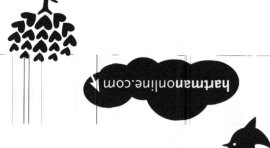

hartmanonline.com

Hartman

Workbook for
Nursing Assisting
A Foundation in Caregiving

FOURTH EDITION

Credits

Managing Editor
Susan Alvare Hedman

Cover Designer
Kirsten Browne

Cover Illustrator
Jo Tronc

Interior Illustrator
Thad Castillo

Production
Thad Castillo

Proofreader
Kristin Cartwright

Copyright Information

© 2016 by Hartman Publishing, Inc.
1313 Iron Ave SW
Albuquerque, New Mexico 87102
(505) 291-1274
web: hartmanonline.com
e-mail: orders@hartmanonline.com
Twitter: @HartmanPub

ISBN 978-1-60425-062-6

PRINTED IN THE USA

Notice to Readers

Though the guidelines and procedures contained in this text are based on consultations with healthcare professionals, they should not be considered absolute recommendations. The instructor and readers should follow employer, local, state, and federal guidelines concerning healthcare practices. These guidelines change, and it is the reader's responsibility to be aware of these changes and of the policies and procedures of her or his healthcare facility.

The publisher, author, editors, and reviewers cannot accept any responsibility for errors or omissions or for any consequences from application of the information in this book and make no warranty, express or implied, with respect to the contents of the book. The publisher does not warrant or guarantee any of the products described herein or perform any analysis in connection with any of the product information contained herein.

Gender Usage

This workbook utilizes the pronouns *he, his, she,* and *her* interchangeably to denote healthcare team members and residents.

Table of Contents

vi

1

The Nursing Assistant in Long-Term Care

1. Review the key terms in Learning Objective 1 before completing the workbook exercises

2. Describe healthcare settings

Multiple Choice
Circle the letter of the answer that best completes the statement or answers the question.

1. Another name for a long-term care (LTC) facility is a(n)
   (A) Nursing home
   (B) Home health facility
   (C) Assisted living facility
   (D) Adult day services apartment

2. A person who lives in a long-term care facility is called a *resident* because
   (A) The facility is her home
   (B) She is picked up at the end of each day to go home
   (C) She does not have any living family members
   (D) She does not need skilled care

3. Assisted living facilities are usually for
   (A) Residents who need around-the-clock intensive care
   (B) Residents who are generally independent and do not need skilled care
   (C) Residents who will die within six months
   (D) Residents who require acute care

4. How does home health aide care differ from nursing assistant care?
   (A) Home health aides do not assist with personal care.
   (B) Home health aides may clean the home and do laundry.
   (C) Home health aides do not have supervisors.
   (D) Home health care takes place in a hospital, rather than in a long-term care facility.

5. A program of care given by a specialist or a team of specialists to restore or improve function after an illness or injury is called
   (A) Acute care
   (B) Subacute care
   (C) Rehabilitation
   (D) Hospice care

6. Inter-generational care is
   (A) People of the same generation spending time together
   (B) Pets brought into a long-term care facility to help brighten a resident's day
   (C) Adult and child care merged so that young and old can spend time together
   (D) The generation caring for children and aging parents at the same time

3. Explain Medicare and Medicaid

True or False
Mark each statement with either a T for true or an F for false.

1. ____ Medicare is a health insurance program for people who are 65 years of age or older.

2. _____ No one younger than 65 is covered by Medicare.

3. _____ Medicare will pay for any services requested by the resident.

4. _____ A person with limited income might qualify for Medicaid.

5. _____ Medicare and Medicaid pay a fixed amount for services based on residents' needs.

4. Describe the residents in long-term care facilities

True or False

1. _____ It is more important for nursing assistants to know each resident individually than to know general facts about most residents.

2. _____ Most residents living in long-term care facilities are male.

3. _____ Residents with the longest average stay in a healthcare facility are residents admitted for terminal care.

4. _____ Dementia is not a common cause of admission to a long-term care facility.

5. _____ Poor health is not the only reason residents are admitted to long-term care facilities. Often they are admitted due to lack of a support system.

6. _____ Lack of outside support is one reason to care for the whole person instead of only the illness or disease.

5. Describe the nursing assistant's role

Short Answer

Answer each of the following questions in the space provided.

1. What are activities of daily living (ADLs)?

_____

_____

_____

_____

2. Think of one task that might be assigned to a nursing assistant that is not mentioned in the book.

_____

_____

_____

_____

_____

3. Look at the tasks commonly performed by nursing assistants. Which task do you think you will enjoy the most? Which do you think will be the most difficult for you?

_____

_____

_____

_____

_____

_____

_____

_____

_____

_____

6. Discuss professionalism and list examples of professional behavior

Multiple Choice

1. Which of the following best shows professionalism by a nursing assistant?
   (A) A nursing assistant arrives late for her shift, knowing her coworkers can cover for her.
   (B) A nursing assistant takes a while to document carefully.
   (C) A nursing assistant uses profanity sometimes, but only if a resident does it first.
   (D) A nursing assistant accepts a tip from a resident's son for taking care of his mother.

2. Katie is a new nursing assistant at Parkwood Skilled Nursing Care and wants to make a positive first impression. Which of the following would be the best way for Katie to demonstrate professionalism at her new job?
   (A) She can avoid asking questions so as not to bother her supervisors.
   (B) She can tell a resident about another resident's condition in order to gain the resident's trust.
   (C) She can avoid unnecessary work absences.
   (D) She can address residents by using affectionate nicknames like "Sweetie."

7. List qualities that nursing assistants must have

Scenarios
Read each of the following scenarios and answer the questions that follow.

Nursing assistant Samantha Stevens is late for five shifts in a row. On the fifth day, her supervisor asks her about this. Samantha replies, "It's not my fault. Traffic has been horrible, and I have to drive a long time to get to work."

1. How could Samantha have been more humble and open to growth?

_____
_____
_____
_____
_____
_____

Nurse Frederico Gonzalez tells nursing assistant Mary Lupko about a resident's diagnosis of a sexually-transmitted infection. He gives specific instructions about the resident's care. Mary sees a fellow nursing assistant across the hall, and says, "How did Joann Timbly get an STI? Her husband hasn't visited in months."

2. How could Mary have been more trustworthy?

_____

_____
_____
_____
_____
_____
_____

Nursing assistant Rob Brown is tidying Ms. Lee's room. He notices a Buddha statue and asks, "I'm a Christian. Why don't you believe in Christ?"

3. How could Rob have acted in a courteous and respectful manner?

_____
_____
_____
_____
_____

Resident Hannah Stein is dying. She tells nursing assistant Jennifer Wells that she always wanted to be nicer to her son and to have a better relationship. Jennifer replies, "Well my son won't even talk to me because I wouldn't let him go to a basketball game on a school night." Then Jennifer proceeds to tell Mrs. Stein about her divorce and how her son's father never helps out.

4. How could Jennifer have been more empathetic?

_____
_____
_____
_____
_____
_____
_____
_____

2. The _____
will usually be the nursing assistant's immediate supervisor.

3. When a nursing assistant has a problem
with another department, it should be
reported to an immediate supervisor or the
_____ nurse.

4. Following the chain of command helps protect staff from
_____, which
is a legal term for being held responsible for
harming someone else.

11. Explain *The Five Rights of Delegation*

Short Answer

1. What are three questions nurses consider
before delegating a task?

_____
_____
_____
_____
_____
_____
_____
_____
_____
_____
_____
_____

2. What are three questions nursing assistants
should ask themselves before accepting a
delegation?

_____
_____
_____
_____

_____
_____
_____
_____
_____

3. If a nursing assistant is unsure about a task
that is delegated to him, what should he do?

_____
_____
_____
_____
_____

12. Describe methods of nursing care and discuss person-centered care

Matching
Use each letter only once.

1. ____ Functional nursing

2. ____ Person-centered care

3. ____ Primary nursing

4. ____ Team nursing

(A) Method of care that revolves around the resident and promotes each individual's preferences, choices, dignity and interests

(B) Method of care in which a nurse acts as the
team leader of the group giving care

(C) Method of care in which each member of
the care team is given specific tasks to perform for a large number of residents

(D) Method of care in which the registered
nurse gives much of the daily care to
residents

13. Explain policy and procedure manuals

Fill in the Blank

1. A _____
is a course of action to be taken every time a
certain situation occurs.

2. A complete list of every facility policy is found in the _____
_____.

3. A _____
is a specific way of doing something.

4. The exact way to complete every resident procedure is found in the _____
_____.

14. Describe the long-term care survey process

True or False

1. _____ A survey is conducted by a team of professionals to make sure long-term care facilities are following state and federal regulations.

2. _____ If a surveyor asks a nursing assistant a question and the nursing assistant does not know the answer, she should quickly make one up to avoid being cited.

3. _____ Surveyors will interview residents to get their opinions about the care they receive.

4. _____ Membership in the Joint Commission is mandatory for all long-term care facilities.

Name: _____

2
Ethical and Legal Issues

1. Review the key terms in Learning Objective 1 before completing the workbook exercises

2. Define the terms *law*, *ethics*, and *etiquette*

Multiple Choice

1. _____ have to do with the knowledge of right and wrong.
   (A) Ethics
   (B) Civil laws
   (C) Etiquette issues
   (D) Criminal laws

2. Which of the following is a law?
   (A) A nursing assistant must not gossip about residents or other staff members.
   (B) A nursing assistant must be polite when answering the telephone.
   (C) A nursing assistant must not steal residents' belongings.
   (D) A nursing assistant must not discuss personal problems with coworkers.

3. Laws to protect individuals from people or organizations that try to harm them are
   (A) Civil laws
   (B) Criminal laws
   (C) Felonies
   (D) Misdemeanors

4. A code of courtesy and proper behavior in a certain setting is called
   (A) Civil law
   (B) Criminal law
   (C) Ethics
   (D) Etiquette

3. Discuss examples of ethical and professional behavior

Crossword Puzzle

Across

1. Treating residents with this means allowing others to believe or act as they wish to do

2. Being able to share in and understand the feelings of others

5. Another word for private

6. Nursing assistants must refuse these when they are offered

Down

1. If a nursing assistant makes a mistake, it is important to do this immediately

3. Being this way means that a nursing assistant is able to speak and act without offending others

4. Ways that a nursing assistant can demonstrate being _____ include being truthful when reporting hours and documenting care accurately

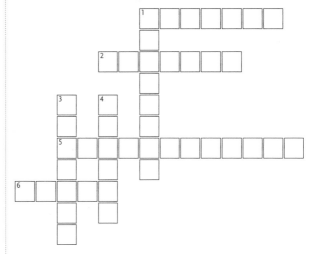

9. Rights during transfers and discharges

_____

_____

_____

_____

_____

_____

10. The right to complain

_____

_____

_____

_____

_____

11. The right to visits

_____

_____

_____

_____

_____

_____

12. Rights with regard to social services

_____

_____

_____

_____

_____

_____

7. Explain types of abuse and neglect

Matching
Use each letter only once.

1. _____ Abuse

2. _____ Active neglect

3. _____ Assault

4. _____ Battery

5. _____ Defamation

6. _____ Domestic violence

7. _____ False imprisonment

8. _____ Financial abuse

9. _____ Involuntary seclusion

10. _____ Libel

11. _____ Malpractice

12. _____ Negligence

13. _____ Passive neglect

14. _____ Physical abuse

15. _____ Psychological abuse

16. _____ Sexual abuse

17. _____ Sexual harassment

18. _____ Slander

19. _____ Substance abuse

20. _____ Verbal abuse

21. _____ Workplace violence

(A) Actions, or the failure to act or provide proper care for a person, resulting in unintended injury

(B) The repeated use of legal or illegal drugs, cigarettes, or alcohol in a way that is harmful to oneself or others

(C) Any unwelcome sexual advance or behavior that creates an intimidating, hostile, or offensive working environment

(D) Purposeful failure to provide needed care, resulting in physical, mental, or emotional harm to a person

(E) The separation of a person from others against the person's will

(F) Unlawful restraint that affects a person's freedom of movement

(G) Verbal, physical, or sexual abuse of staff by other staff members, residents, or visitors

(H) The intentional touching of a person without his or her consent

(I) A threat to harm a person, resulting in the person feeling fearful that he or she will be harmed

(J) Improper or illegal use of a person's money, possessions, property, or other assets

(K) Any statement that is not true that injures a person's reputation

(L) The forcing of unwanted sexual acts or behavior on a person

(M) The use of language that threatens, embarrasses, or insults a person

(N) Emotional harm caused by threatening, frightening, isolating, intimidating, humiliating, or insulting a person

(O) Physical, sexual, or emotional abuse by spouses, intimate partners, or family members

(P) Purposeful mistreatment that causes physical, mental, emotional, or financial pain or injury to a person

(Q) Any treatment, intentional or unintentional, that causes harm to a person's body

(R) Unintentional failure to provide needed care, resulting in physical, mental, or emotional harm to a person

(S) Defamation in written form

(T) Defamation in oral form

(U) Professional misconduct that results in damage or injury to a person

Multiple Choice

1. What should a nursing assistant do if he sees or suspects that a resident is being abused?
   (A) The NA should report it to the supervisor and document it at once.
   (B) The NA should keep watching the resident until he is sure he is correct.
   (C) The NA should ignore it unless the resident complains about it.
   (D) The NA should confront the abuser immediately.

2. If a resident wants to make a complaint of abuse, the nursing assistant's responsibility is to
   (A) Investigate that the abuse has really occurred
   (B) Assist the resident in every possible way
   (C) Counsel the resident to help him or her get over the abuse
   (D) Ask other residents if they have seen any abuse occurring

3. An example of sexual abuse is
   (A) A nursing assistant ignores a resident's call light
   (B) A nursing assistant shows a resident a pornographic magazine
   (C) A nursing assistant leaves a resident alone in his room and does not check on him
   (D) A nursing assistant screams at a resident

4. An example of financial abuse is
   (A) A nursing assistant loudly announces in the hallway that a resident has "wet his bed again"
   (B) A nursing assistant makes fun of a resident's religion
   (C) A nursing assistant receives money from a resident to get a faster response time when the resident calls
   (D) A nursing assistant hits a resident when the resident yells at him

5. An example of psychological abuse is
   (A) A nursing assistant pushes a resident to get to the bathroom more quickly
   (B) A nursing assistant tells a resident he needs money for school
   (C) A nursing assistant forces a resident to rub up against her
   (D) While giving care to a resident, a nursing assistant tells him he smells bad

8. Recognize signs and symptoms of abuse and neglect

True or False

1. _____ Ignoring a call light is not considered abuse or neglect.

2. _____ Broken bones, burns, and bruising are all possible signs of abuse.

3. _____ Weight loss can be a sign of neglect.

4. _____ Similar injuries that occur repeatedly probably just mean that the resident is clumsy.

5. _____ If a resident shows fear or anxiety when a certain caregiver is present, this may be a sign of abuse.

6. _____ Mood swings and depression are always caused by illness or chemical imbalance.

7. _____ If a resident is not clean or smells like urine, it probably just means he does not like to bathe.

8. _____ Pressure ulcers on a resident's body can indicate neglect.

9. _____ If a resident's family is concerned that abuse is occurring, it is considered a possible sign of abuse.

10. _____ If a nursing assistant only suspects abuse, she should wait until she is sure it is happening before reporting it.

9. Describe the steps taken if a nursing assistant is suspected of abuse

Multiple Choice

1. What is the first thing that normally happens when a report of nursing assistant abuse has been made?
   (A) The NA is fired.
   (B) The NA is suspended.
   (C) The NA is taken into custody.
   (D) The NA is transferred to another facility until the investigation is completed.

2. Which of the following is a step taken after a claim of abuse against a nursing assistant has been made?
   (A) An investigation is performed.
   (B) The nursing assistant is charged with a crime.
   (C) The resident is relocated to another facility.
   (D) The facility is closed to the public.

3. If the claim of abuse is proven to be true, what happens?
   (A) The NA is placed in the abuse registry in addition to other possible penalties.
   (B) The resident is moved to another facility.
   (C) The NA is transferred to another facility in another state.
   (D) The facility is cited for negligence.

10. Discuss the ombudsman's role

Short Answer

1. What is the role of an ombudsman?

_____

_____

_____

_____

_____

_____

_____

_____

_____

_____

_____

2. Which other people or organizations can a resident or his family contact for help or to make a complaint?

_____

_____

_____

_____

_____

_____

11. Explain HIPAA and related terms

Multiple Choice

1. Why was the Health Insurance Portability and Accountability Act (HIPAA) created?
    (A) To protect the privacy of health information
    (B) To reduce instances of abuse in facilities
    (C) To address infection prevention issues in facilities
    (D) To ensure that elderly people have health insurance

2. What is included under a person's private health information (PHI)?
    (A) The person's activity preferences
    (B) The person's social security number
    (C) The person's favorite food
    (D) The person's favorite color

3. What is the correct response by a nursing assistant if someone who is not directly involved with a resident's care asks for a resident's PHI?
    (A) The NA should report the request to the resident.
    (B) The NA should ask the resident's family if it is okay to share the information.
    (C) The NA should tell them that the information is confidential and cannot be given.
    (D) The NA should give the person the information.

4. Which of the following is a way to keep private health information confidential?
    (A) Discussing a resident's care with a coworker in a restaurant
    (B) Posting information on Twitter
    (C) Only discussing residents with family or friends
    (D) Logging out or exiting the web browser when finished with computer work

5. Which of the following is considered an invasion of a resident's privacy?
    (A) A nursing assistant tells her supervisor that she thinks a resident is starting to develop a pressure ulcer.
    (B) A nursing assistant shows her husband a photo of a new resident in her care.
    (C) A nursing assistant documents a resident's complaint of pain.
    (D) A nursing assistant refuses to share information about a resident with the resident's sister.

6. The abbreviation for a law that was enacted as a part of the American Recovery and Reinvestment Act of 2009 and helps expand the protection and security of consumers' electronic health records (EHR) is called
    (A) HISEAL
    (B) HITECH
    (C) HIHELP
    (D) HIQUIET

12. Discuss the Patient Self-Determination Act (PSDA) and advance directives

True or False

1. ____ A DNR order tells healthcare professionals to keep trying to resuscitate a resident in the event of cardiac arrest.

2. ____ The Patient Self-Determination Act is meant to encourage people to make decisions about advance directives.

3. ____ Advance directives designate the kind of care people want in the event they are unable to make those decisions themselves.

4. ____ A living will designates the people who will inherit the resident's estate when he or she dies.

5. ____ A durable power of attorney for health care appoints a person to make medical decisions for a resident in the event he or she becomes unable to do so.

6. ____ Facilities are required by Medicare and Medicaid to give residents and staff information about rights relating to advance directives.

3

Communication Skills

1. Review the key terms in Learning Objective 1 before completing the workbook exercises

2. Explain types of communication

True or False

1. ____ People communicate with words, drawings, pictures, and behavior.

2. ____ The receiver and sender do not switch roles as they communicate.

3. ____ Speaking and writing are two examples of verbal communication.

4. ____ How a person's voice sounds and the words he chooses are not important during communication.

5. ____ Nonverbal communication includes posture and facial expressions.

6. ____ Making positive changes in body language will improve communication.

7. ____ A nursing assistant can be helpful by finishing a resident's sentences to show that she understands what he is telling her.

8. ____ The nursing assistant should use mostly facts when communicating with the care team.

Short Answer

State whether each behavior is an example of positive or negative nonverbal communication. Write "P" for positive or "N" for negative.

1. ____ Smiling

2. ____ Crossing arms in front of the body

3. ____ Looking away while someone is talking

4. ____ Leaning forward in a chair

5. ____ Pointing at someone while speaking

6. ____ Rolling eyes

7. ____ Putting a hand over a resident's hand

8. ____ Tapping a foot

9. ____ Nodding while a person is speaking

3. Explain barriers to communication

Scenarios

Read the scenarios below and answer the questions.

Nursing assistant Barbara Smith thinks resident Mrs. Gold is in pain. Barbara asks her if she is okay. Before Mrs. Gold answers, Barbara looks around the room and begins to gather her supplies to leave. Mrs. Gold simply says, "Yes."

1. Identify the barrier to communication occurring here and suggest a way to avoid it.

_____

_____

_____

_____

_____

_____

_____

_____

_____

_____

_____

_____

Communication Skills

Resident Marla Gibson had a stroke that affects her speech. She asks her nursing assistant for a glass of water. The nursing assistant replies, "I'm not sure where your daughter is," and leaves the room.

2. Identify the barrier to communication occurring here and suggest a way to avoid it.

_____
_____
_____
_____
_____
_____
_____
_____
_____

Nursing assistant Kena Wright asks resident Josiah Crane, "You are NWB, right?" He nods. She reports to the nurse, who says, "That is not true. He is allowed to bear full weight on both legs."

3. Identify the barrier to communication occurring here and suggest a way to avoid it.

_____
_____
_____
_____
_____
_____
_____
_____
_____
_____
_____
_____

Nursing assistant Jerry Wells sees that resident Eli Levine is having difficulty moving his leg after his total hip replacement surgery. Jerry says, "I've helped many residents after this type of surgery. You should start doing exercises right away and begin bearing as much weight as possible." Mr. Levine attempts to stand on his leg and yells in pain.

4. Identify the barrier to communication occurring here and suggest a way to avoid it.

_____
_____
_____
_____
_____
_____
_____
_____
_____

Resident Paul Jackson is at risk for dehydration. Nursing assistants are asked to encourage him to drink as much as possible. To find out what Mr. Jackson likes to drink, nursing assistant Gracie Truman asks him, "Do you like orange juice?" He says, "No."

5. Identify the barrier to communication occurring here and suggest a way to avoid it.

_____
_____
_____
_____
_____
_____
_____
_____
_____
_____

Nursing assistant Lyla Cooper is helping resident Josie Bayer get ready to attend a guest lecture with another resident. Josie says, "I don't want to go with her." Lyla asks, "Why not?" Josie replies, "I just don't."

6. Identify the barrier to communication occurring here and suggest a way to avoid it.

_____

_____

_____

_____

_____

_____

_____

_____

Nursing assistant Tracy Fleming is assigned to give Mr. Perez, who speaks very little English, a bed bath. She explains the procedure, and Mr. Perez nods even though he looks a little confused. When she starts to take off his shirt, he gets very upset.

7. Identify the barrier to communication occurring here and suggest a way to avoid it.

_____

_____

_____

_____

_____

_____

_____

_____

4. List ways that cultures impact communication

Multiple Choice

1. Which of the following is true of cultures?
   (A) There are only a few cultures in the world.
   (B) The use of touch is the same for all cultures.
   (C) A culture is a set of learned beliefs, values, and behaviors.
   (D) The use of eye contact is the same for all cultures.

2. If a resident seems to be sensitive to eye contact and/or touch, a nursing assistant should
   (A) Make eye contact and touch him as much as possible so that the resident is able to get used to it
   (B) Respect his wishes and limit eye contact and touch as much as possible
   (C) Explain to the resident that in the United States things are done differently and he should start adapting
   (D) Ignore the sensitivity and use eye contact and touch as with any other resident

3. Which of the following is a type of unacceptable touch by an NA when working with a resident?
   (A) Sitting on the resident's lap
   (B) Cleaning the resident's arm during a bed bath
   (C) Hugging the resident
   (D) Holding the resident's hand

4. One appropriate way for a nursing assistant to deal with a language barrier with a resident is to
   (A) Use an interpreter
   (B) Teach the resident words in the NA's language
   (C) Speak with other staff in the NA's language in front of the resident
   (D) Get someone else to care for the resident

5. Identify the people a nursing assistant communicates with in a facility

True or False

1. _____ When a nursing assistant first greets a resident, he should introduce himself and identify the resident.

2. _____ In the facility, a nursing assistant may communicate by charting, using a computer, or on the telephone.

3. _____ If a nursing assistant has performed a procedure for a resident before, she does not need to explain it the next time she does it.

4. _____ Communication with other departments within a facility is not common and is unimportant.

5. _____ One way to let a resident's family know that staff are providing proper care for him is to always answer call lights promptly.

6. _____ Families can provide valuable information about a resident's preferences and histories.

7. _____ If a staff member from a doctor's office calls and asks for information about a resident, the nursing assistant should give it to her.

6. Understand basic medical terminology and abbreviations

Matching
For each of the following abbreviations, write the letter of the correct term from the list below. Use each letter only once.

1. _____ ADLs

2. _____ amb

3. _____ BM

4. _____ c/o

5. _____ DNR

6. _____ DX, dx

7. _____ f/u, F/U

8. _____ inc

9. _____ I&O

10. _____ NPO

11. _____ mL

12. _____ prn, PRN

13. _____ ROM

14. _____ vs, VS

15. _____ w/c, W/C

(A) Diagnosis

(B) Incontinent

(C) Activities of daily living

(D) Nothing by mouth

(E) Bowel movement

(F) Do not resuscitate

(G) Complains of

(H) Range of motion

(I) Vital signs

(J) Wheelchair

(K) As necessary

(L) Intake and output

(M) Milliliter

(N) Follow up

(O) Ambulate

7. Explain how to convert regular time to military time

Short Answer

Convert the following times to military time:

1. 2:10 p.m. _____

2. 4:30 a.m. _____

3. 10:00 a.m. _____

4. 8:25 p.m. _____

Convert the following times to regular time:

5. 0600 _____

6. 2320 _____

7. 1927 _____

8. 1800 _____

8. Describe a standard resident chart

Multiple Choice

1. When charting, the nursing assistant's role is limited to which of the following?
   (A) Making changes in residents' diets
   (B) Changing medications when current ones are not working
   (C) Gathering information and reporting to the nurse
   (D) Creating a new exercise plan

2. Which of the following is true of a resident's medical chart?
   (A) The nursing assistant includes her qualifications in the medical chart.
   (B) Nursing assistants write their diagnoses in the medical chart.
   (C) Information about the resident's roommate is included in the medical chart.
   (D) Nurses' notes are included in the medical chart.

9. Explain guidelines for documentation

Multiple Choice

1. If a mistake is made when charting care, the best response by the nursing assistant would be to
   (A) Erase what she has written and enter the correct information
   (B) Draw a line through the error and initial and date it
   (C) Use white correction fluid to cross out the error and then initial and date the white area
   (D) Staple a new sheet to the front of the medical chart that has the correct information

2. When is it appropriate for an NA to chart care before it has been done?
   (A) When a resident requests it
   (B) Never
   (C) When the NA will not have time afterward to do it
   (D) When a procedure will take a long time

3. What color of ink is the best choice for documenting by hand?
   (A) Red
   (B) Black
   (C) Blue
   (D) Green

4. Which statement below is an example of a fact?
   (A) Ms. Lopez was grumpy at dinner.
   (B) Ms. Lopez did not like the chicken.
   (C) Ms. Lopez ate all of her vegetables.
   (D) Ms. Lopez became depressed while eating.

10. Describe the use of computers in documentation

Fill in the Blank

1. Computers can easily store information that can be _____ when needed.

2. Using a computer for charting is faster and more _____ than writing by hand.

3. In some facilities a _____ or tablet is moved from room to room to document care.

4. An NA should not share his personal _____ with anyone.

5. An NA should not access _____ e-mail accounts or view inappropriate _____ from work.

6. _____ privacy guidelines apply to computer use.

11. Explain the Minimum Data Set (MDS)

Multiple Choice

1. The Minimum Data Set (MDS) was created to
   (A) Give facilities a standardized approach to care
   (B) Give facilities more flexibility in how care is performed
   (C) Improve infection prevention methods in facilities
   (D) Help train nursing assistants how to do particular care procedures

2. For which of the following situations does an MDS need to be completed?
   (A) When a resident leaves the facility
   (B) Once every five years after the first MDS has been completed
   (C) When there have been no major changes in a resident's condition for two weeks
   (D) Within 14 days of a resident's admission

3. What is the nursing assistant's role regarding the MDS?
   (A) Completing the MDS for each resident
   (B) Reminding the nurse when the MDS needs to be done
   (C) Reporting changes in residents' health
   (D) Deciding how to address problems discovered in the assessment

12. Describe how to observe and report accurately

True or False

1. _____ Nursing assistants may notice more changes in residents than other care team members because they spend the most time with residents.

2. _____ Changes in a resident's condition that endanger residents should be reported right away.

3. _____ Nursing assistants make decisions regarding residents' health.

4. _____ Critical thinking for nursing assistants means the ability to make careful observations.

5. _____ A care plan is a plan for each resident that outlines the steps and tasks needed to help the resident achieve her goals of care.

6. _____ Care plans are developed by nursing assistants.

7. _____ Changes in a resident's weight do not need to be reported unless they are over 10 pounds.

Short Answer

For each of the following, decide whether it is an objective observation (you can see, hear, smell, or touch it) or subjective observation (the resident must tell you about it). Write "O" for objective and "S" for subjective.

1. _____ Skin rash

2. _____ Crying

3. _____ Rapid pulse

4. _____ Headache

5. _____ Nausea

6. _____ Vomiting

7. _____ Swelling

8. _____ Cloudy urine

9. _____ Wheezing

10. _____ Feeling sad

11. _____ Red area on skin

12. _____ Fever

13. _____ Dizziness

14. _____ Chest pain

15. _____ Toothache

16. _____ Coughing

17. _____ Fruity breath

18. _____ Itchy arm

Short Answer

19. For each of these four senses, list two observations that a nursing assistant might make using that sense.

- Sight

  _____

  _____

  _____

  _____

- Hearing

  _____

  _____

  _____

  _____

- Touch

  _____

  _____

  _____

  _____

- Smell

  _____

  _____

  _____

  _____

13. Explain the nursing process

Matching
Use each letter only once.

1. ____ Assessment

2. ____ Diagnosis

3. ____ Evaluation

4. ____ Implementation

5. ____ Planning

(A) In agreement with the resident, goals are set and a care plan is created to meet the resident's needs

(B) A careful examination to see if goals were met or progress was achieved

(C) Getting information from many sources to identify actual and potential problems

(D) Putting the care plan into action; giving care

(E) The identification of health problems after looking at all of the resident's needs

14. Discuss the nursing assistant's role in care planning and at care conferences

Multiple Choice

1. The purpose of a care conference is to
   (A) Train nursing assistants in new care skills
   (B) Decide how to remove a resident from a facility
   (C) Share information about residents to develop a plan of care
   (D) Orient new residents to the facility

2. What is the nursing assistant's role at a care conference?
   (A) The NA keeps order at the meeting.
   (B) The NA shares resident observations.
   (C) The NA suggests any new medications that might be beneficial for the resident.
   (D) The NA explains the care plan to the resident and his family.

3. If a nursing assistant is not sure what to say at a care conference, she should
   (A) Not attend the conference
   (B) Attend the conference but check with the resident's family about what she can share
   (C) Talk to the nurse before the conference to find out what she should say
   (D) Ask other nursing assistants at the meeting what information she should share

15. Describe incident reporting and recording

Multiple Choice

1. Which of the following would be considered an incident?
    (A) A resident is acting withdrawn.
    (B) A resident accuses a staff member of abuse.
    (C) A resident returns from a family outing later than she said she would be.
    (D) A resident tells a staff member that she does not like her roommate.

2. Documenting an incident and the response to the incident is done in a(n)
    (A) Minimum Data Set report
    (B) Flow sheet report
    (C) Incident report
    (D) Sentinel report

3. Which of the following is something that the NA should include when documenting an incident?
    (A) Facts regarding what the NA saw
    (B) Opinions of why the incident occurred
    (C) Suggestions for changes in the resident's care
    (D) Ideas for revising how incident reports are completed

16. Explain proper telephone etiquette

Multiple Choice

1. An example of proper telephone etiquette is
    (A) Immediately putting the caller on hold without asking
    (B) Identifying the facility to the caller
    (C) Letting the caller know when it is not a good time to call
    (D) Giving the caller any information about residents and staff she needs

2. Which of the following is a general rule for telephone use at a facility?
    (A) All facilities allow the use of cell phones at work.
    (B) Staff information can be disclosed to creditors if they call.
    (C) Resident information can be given to anyone who calls and inquires.
    (D) Resident information cannot be given over the phone.

17. Describe the resident call system

Short Answer

1. What is the purpose of the facility call system?

    _____

    _____

    _____

    _____

    _____

    _____

    _____

2. Why is answering a resident's call light promptly so important?

    _____

    _____

    _____

    _____

    _____

    _____

    _____

    _____

18. Describe the nursing assistant's role in change-of-shift reports and rounds

Fill in the Blank

1. Examples of information passed on to the next shift are _____ that occurred, appetite problems, difficulties with urination, complaints of _____, or a change in the ability to _____.

2. At start of shift reports, the NA should listen to important information about all of the _____ in the area.

3. Special information shared during a report may include new _____ and transfers or _____ from the facility.

4. Before the end of shift report, the NA should tell the nurses about such things as changes in _____ or temperature and skin changes that could signal the start of a _____.

5. A method of reporting where staff members move from room to room and discuss each resident and the plan of care is called _____.

19. List the information found on an assignment sheet

Matching

1. _____ Activities of daily living

2. _____ Code

3. _____ Code status

4. _____ Range of motion

(A) Exercises done to bring joints through a full range of movement

(B) Explains the type of care that should be provided to a resident in the event of a cardiac arrest, other catastrophic organ failure, or terminal illness

(C) Tasks that are done for residents every day

(D) An emergent medical situation in which specially-trained responders provide the necessary care

20. Discuss how to organize work and manage time

Crossword Puzzle
Across

4. Talking with residents while providing care is an example of _____ activities

5. Identifying the most important things to get done and doing those first

6. Being able to ask for this when needed is important

Down

1. Should be within a resident's reach before a nursing assistant leaves him

2. Doing this with work helps nursing assistants complete their assignments each day

3. Making one of these involves writing out the hours of the day and filling in when a nursing assistant will do what

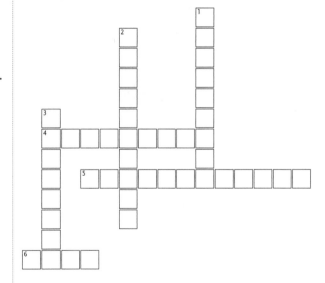

Name: _____

4

Communication Challenges

1. Review the key terms in Learning Objective 1 before completing the workbook exercises

2. Identify communication guidelines for visual impairment

Multiple Choice

1. A partial or complete loss of function or ability is an
   (A) Imperative
   (B) Impairment
   (C) Infraction
   (D) Infinite

2. One disease that can cause visual impairment is
   (A) Diabetes
   (B) Chronic Obstructive Pulmonary Disease
   (C) Dermatitis
   (D) Irritable Bowel Syndrome

3. What is the first step a nursing assistant should take before touching a resident who is visually impaired?
   (A) The NA should put away the resident's personal items.
   (B) The NA should read the menu.
   (C) The NA should change the resident's sheets.
   (D) The NA should identify herself.

4. What is important for an NA to note about a resident's eyeglasses?
   (A) Whether the eyeglasses are stylish
   (B) Whether the eyeglasses fit properly
   (C) Whether the eyeglasses have glass or plastic lenses
   (D) Whether the lenses darken automatically when exposed to sunlight

5. Which of the following would be the best way for an NA to explain the position of objects to a resident who is visually impaired?
   (A) The NA can take the resident around the room and have her touch items to know where they are located.
   (B) The NA can let the resident know how far objects are from the resident using approximate measurements of inches, feet, and yards.
   (C) The NA can describe the position of objects using the face of an imaginary clock.
   (D) The NA can use the directional terms *north*, *south*, *east*, and *west* to describe the position of objects.

3. Identify communication guidelines for hearing impairment

Multiple Choice

1. Which of the following is a symptom of hearing loss?
   (A) Trouble hearing high-pitched noises
   (B) Trouble hearing vowels
   (C) Being able to understand the meanings of words
   (D) Being able to hear people who are outside of the room

2. Which of the following is the best way for a nursing assistant to communicate with a resident who has a hearing impairment?
   (A) The NA should exaggerate the pronunciation of words.
   (B) The NA should shout when speaking.
   (C) The NA should raise the pitch of her voice.
   (D) The NA should use simple words and short sentences.

Name: _____

4. Explain defense mechanisms as methods of coping with stress

True or False

1. ____ Defense mechanisms allow a person to release tension.

2. ____ Repression means seeing feelings in others that are actually feelings within oneself.

3. ____ Displacement means transferring a strong feeling to a less threatening object.

4. ____ Defense mechanisms help a person face the reasons a situation has occurred.

5. ____ Denial is rejecting a thought or feeling.

6. ____ Regression is making excuses to justify something.

5. List communication guidelines for anxiety or fear

Short Answer

1. Define *anxiety*.

_____

_____

_____

_____

_____

2. List four physical symptoms of anxiety.

_____

_____

_____

_____

_____

_____

_____

3. List five guidelines for communicating with an anxious resident.

_____

_____

_____

_____

_____

_____

_____

6. Discuss communication guidelines for depression

True or False

1. ____ Losses that a resident may be experiencing include the loss of a spouse, friends, and independence.

2. ____ Clinical depression can be managed, but it cannot be cured.

3. ____ One behavior that is associated with clinical depression is a lack of interest in activities.

4. ____ Most people who are depressed could choose to be well if they wanted to.

5. ____ It is never a good idea for a nursing assistant to touch a resident who is depressed.

6. ____ NAs should not talk to adults as if they were children.

7. ____ Depressed residents will never want to talk about their feelings.

8. ____ NAs should report signs of depression right away.

7. Identify communication guidelines for anger

Fill in the Blank

1. _____ is a natural emotion that may be expressed by residents, their families and friends, and staff members.

2. Loss of _____ can cause a resident to be angry.

3. Narrowed _____ and clenched or raised _____ are signs of anger.

4. Anger may also be expressed by withdrawing or being _____.

5. If a resident becomes angry frequently, a _____ may be scheduled.

6. When dealing with an angry resident, the NA should try to find out what _____ the resident's anger.

7. The NA should not _____with an angry resident.

8. The NA can try to involve the resident in _____.

9. Being _____ means being confident in dealing with other people. Being _____ means expressing oneself in a way that humiliates or overpowers another person.

8. Identify communication guidelines for combative behavior

Multiple Choice

1. Which of the following would be the best response by a nursing assistant when a resident is being combative?
   (A) The NA should call for the nurse immediately.
   (B) The NA should stay as close to the resident as she can.
   (C) The NA should respond to insults with humor or sarcasm.
   (D) The NA should threaten the resident if the behavior does not stop.

2. A nursing assistant's responsibility when a resident becomes combative is to
   (A) Leave the resident alone until he is calm
   (B) Let the resident know that he is upsetting everyone and needs to stop
   (C) Keep other people at a safe distance
   (D) Restrain the resident if he does not calm down

3. Under what circumstances may a nursing assistant hit a resident?
   (A) Any time a resident becomes combative
   (B) If the resident threatens to hit the nursing assistant first
   (C) Only if the resident actually hits the nursing assistant
   (D) Never

9. Identify communication guidelines for inappropriate sexual behavior

Crossword Puzzle

Across

2. Nursing assistants must not do this regarding residents' sexual behavior

5. A nursing assistant should not _____ when encountering an embarrassing situation, but instead should remain professional and calm.

6. Touching or rubbing sexual organs in order to give oneself or another person sexual pleasure

Down

1. Removing these in public areas is one example of inappropriate sexual behavior

3. One illness that can cause inappropriate sexual behavior

4. What a nursing assistant should provide if she witnesses consenting adults in a sexual situation

Communication Challenges

Name: _____

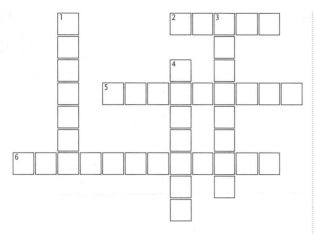

10. Identify communication guidelines for disorientation and confusion

Short Answer

1. Define *disorientation* and *confusion*.

_____

_____

_____

_____

_____

_____

_____

_____

2. List three things that a resident who is oriented should be able to tell the nursing assistant.

_____

_____

_____

_____

_____

_____

_____

_____

3. Name five physical problems that may cause confusion.

_____

_____

_____

_____

_____

_____

_____

_____

_____

4. How can a nursing assistant make tasks easier for a person who is disoriented or confused?

_____

_____

_____

_____

_____

_____

_____

11. Identify communication guidelines for the comatose resident

Multiple Choice

1. Which of the following is true of a resident who is comatose?
   (A) A resident who is comatose is conscious.
   (B) A resident who is comatose can respond to changes in the environment.
   (C) A resident who is comatose may be able to hear what is going on in the room.
   (D) A nursing assistant should avoid speaking to a resident who is comatose.

2. Which of the following should a nursing assistant do when caring for a resident who is comatose?
    (A) The NA should explain each procedure that he will be performing to the resident.
    (B) The NA should avoid announcing when he enters and leaves the room since the resident is not aware of anything.
    (C) The NA should remain silent at all times to avoid disturbing the resident.
    (D) The NA should not touch the resident.

12. Identify communication guidelines for functional barriers

Fill in the Blank

1. Some things that can interfere with the ability to speak include difficulty _____, physical problems with the _____ or _____, or an artificial _____.

2. Birth defects such as cleft _____ may make speech difficult.

3. A(n) _____ is an opening through the neck into the trachea that is surgically created.

4. The resident can _____ anything that is not understood by the NA.

5. The NA should not remove a resident's _____ for any reason.

6. The NA should always report if the resident has poorly fitting _____.

7. The NA should be _____ to the resident's situation by imagining how it might feel to have a tube in the nose, mouth, or throat.

Name: _____

5

Diversity and Human Needs and Development

1. Review the key terms in Learning Objective 1 before completing the workbook exercises

2. Explain health and wellness

Multiple Choice

1. The focus of health should be
   (A) On the whole person
   (B) On the person's diagnosed disease
   (C) On the person's disability
   (D) On the person's poor health habits

2. The types of wellness are
   (A) Physical, social, emotional, intellectual, and ethical
   (B) Physical, social, emotional, financial, and spiritual
   (C) Physical, social, sexual, intellectual, and nutritional
   (D) Physical, social, emotional, intellectual, and spiritual

3. Explain the importance of holistic health care

Multiple Choice

1. Holistic care involves
   (A) Dividing a system into parts
   (B) Caring only for a person's physical needs
   (C) Caring only for a person's psychosocial needs
   (D) Caring for the whole person

2. Which of the following is an example of a psychosocial need?
   (A) Need for food
   (B) Need to nurture spirituality
   (C) Need to be free from pain
   (D) Need for shelter

3. Which of the following is an example of giving holistic care to a resident?
   (A) Asking a resident to talk about her day while giving her a bath
   (B) Rushing a resident through dinner to get tasks done more quickly
   (C) Choosing a resident's clothes for him so he does not have to worry about it
   (D) Trying to convert a resident to the nursing assistant's religion so that they will have something in common

4. Identify basic human needs and discuss Maslow's Hierarchy of Needs

Fill in the Blank

1. A _____ is something necessary for a person to survive and grow.

2. Residents need to feel as if they

   _____

   in their new home.

3. The first needs nursing assistants help residents meet are _____ needs like food and water, rest, and sleep.

4. Moving a person from her home into a facility can cause _____.

5. Residents may feel less of a sense of self-worth as they become

   _____ on others.

6. The highest need a person can achieve, according to Maslow, is _____
_____.

5. Identify ways to accommodate cultural differences

True or False

1. ____ Generally, a nursing assistant will not need to understand different cultures to provide better care to residents.

2. ____ Culture and background do not affect the way people behave when they are ill.

3. ____ A nursing assistant should respond to new ideas with acceptance rather than prejudice.

4. ____ People of all cultures tend to be embarrassed about discussing their health.

5. ____ In the United States, there are only a few different cultures.

6. ____ Cultural competence is an ongoing process of learning about each person's beliefs.

6. Discuss the role of the family in health care

Multiple Choice

1. Which of the following is true of families?
   (A) Some families are the right kind of family, while others are the wrong kind.
   (B) Families play an important role in residents' health care.
   (C) Unmarried couples should not be considered a type of family.
   (D) Families should not be allowed privacy for visits with residents.

2. Which of the following is an example of a nuclear family?
   (A) A mother, a father, and a child
   (B) A mother, a father, a grandfather, and a child
   (C) An uncle, a friend, and one parent
   (D) A cousin, an aunt, and a child

3. Which of the following is the best response by the nursing assistant when a resident has his family visiting?
   (A) The NA should do everything possible to help the resident prepare for the visit.
   (B) The NA should ignore the visitors so as not to bother them.
   (C) The NA should tell the resident's family funny stories about the resident.
   (D) The NA should watch the family closely to make sure the resident is not abused during the visit.

7. Explain how to meet emotional needs of residents and their families

Crossword Puzzle

Across

3. Staff members who are prone to this are at risk for inappropriate relationships with residents

4. The care team member that families should be referred to when they ask nursing assistants about a resident's diagnosis

5. Nursing assistants must maintain these when working with residents and their families

6. An example of this is, "Everything will be fine" or, "It all works out in the end."

Down

1. Nursing assistants can answer questions asked by residents and their families as long as the questions are within the NA's
   _____

2. It is important that nursing assistants listen and not do this when residents go to them with their problems

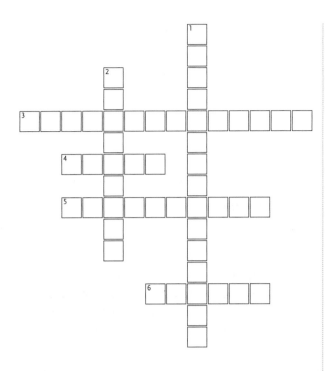

5. _____ Hinduism

6. _____ Islam

7. _____ Judaism

(A) The Five Pillars of this religion include ritual prayer five times daily and donations to the poor and needy

(B) Baptism and communion may be part of this religion's practices

(C) Believe that they do not know or cannot know if God exists

(D) Believe that a person can reach Nirvana, the highest spiritual plane, after traveling through birth, life, and death

(E) Believe that how a person moves toward enlightenment is determined by karma (the result of actions in this life and past lives that can determine one's destiny in future lives)

(F) Believe that God gave them laws and commandments through Moses in the form of the Torah

(G) Actively deny the existence of any deity (higher power)

8. Explain ways to help residents with their spiritual needs

True or False

1. _____ A resident's religious items must be handled carefully.

2. _____ Respecting religious beliefs includes letting Muslim residents know about Christianity.

3. _____ Spiritual needs are different for each person.

4. _____ Some people consider themselves spiritual but do not believe in a higher power.

5. _____ Residents who do not believe in God will not feel as strongly about this belief as residents who do.

Matching
Write the letter of the correct description beside each term related to religious faith or belief. Use each letter only once.

1. _____ Agnosticism

2. _____ Atheism

3. _____ Buddhism

4. _____ Christianity

9. Identify ways to accommodate sexual needs

Matching
Use each letter only once.

1. _____ Asexual

2. _____ Bisexual

3. _____ Celibate

4. _____ Cross-dresser

5. _____ Gay

6. _____ Heterosexual

7. _____ Lesbian

8. _____ LGBT

9. _____ Transgender

10. _____ Transition

Name: _____

(A) The process of changing genders; can include legal procedures, such as changing one's name and/or sex on documents, and medical measures, such as hormone therapy and surgery

(B) A person who abstains from sexual activity

(C) A person whose physical, emotional, and/or romantic attraction is for people of the same sex

(D) Typically a heterosexual man who sometimes wears clothing and other items associated with women

(E) A person whose gender identity conflicts with his or her birth sex

(F) A person whose physical, emotional, and/or romantic attraction is for people of the same gender or another gender

(G) A person whose physical, emotional, and/or romantic attraction is for people of the opposite sex

(H) Acronym for lesbian, gay, bisexual, and transgender

(I) A woman whose physical, emotional, and/or romantic attraction is for other women

(J) A person who does not experience sexual attraction toward any gender

Short Answer

1. Gilda and Samantha both live in a care facility. Gilda is widowed, and Samantha has never been married. They met when Gilda was admitted six months ago. Gilda and Samantha have been sitting at the same table to eat their meals since Gilda moved in. Recently they have started spending time watching TV and playing cards in the day room together. Yesterday they took a walk outside. Linda, a nursing assistant, was gazing out the window and noticed them holding hands. Then she saw them stop behind the building and share a quick kiss. What are some responses that would respect Samantha's and Gilda's dignity and rights?

_____

_____

2. Mr. Ramirez has a private room. His wife lives quite a distance away and only visits once every two weeks. The last time she visited, she requested a dinner tray and asked for both meals to be brought to his room. When Linda went to his room to deliver the meals, the door was shut. She walked in without knocking, and found them kissing each other in bed. She quickly exited the room and almost dropped the food on her way out. What could Linda have done differently? What should she do now that there has been an embarrassing moment?

_____

_____

_____

_____

_____

_____

_____

_____

3. What are two reasons for a lack of sexual expression in long-term care facilities?

_____

_____

_____

_____

10. Describe the stages of human growth and development

Fill in the Blank

1. _____ refers to physical changes that can be measured.

2. _____ means the emotional, social, and physical changes that occur in a person's life.

3. _____ development is the process of gaining an ability to do such things as walking, drawing, and grasping.

4. _____ development is the process of children forming a sense of right and wrong.

5. _____ development focuses on how children think and learn.

6. _____ development is the process of learning to relate to other people.

7. _____ development has to do with the reproductive changes that occur when young people reach puberty.

Multiple Choice

1. In which stage of development is playing dress-up in parents' clothing common?
   (A) Toddler
   (B) Preschool
   (C) Adolescence
   (D) Infancy

2. Both genders become fully sexually mature during this stage of development:
   (A) School-age
   (B) Adolescence
   (C) Middle adulthood
   (D) Late adulthood

3. Decisions about education, employment, and marriage often occur during this stage:
   (A) Young adulthood
   (B) Preadolescence
   (C) Late adulthood
   (D) Adolescence

4. Which of the following is true of late adulthood?
   (A) People no longer need to stay connected to others.
   (B) People in this stage do not need to remain active.
   (C) People often retire from jobs and may need more medical care.
   (D) People undergo very few changes during this stage of life.

11. Discuss stereotypes of the elderly

Multiple Choice

1. Making a biased generalization based on distorted ideas about a group is
   (A) Stereotyping
   (B) Exaggerating
   (C) Opining
   (D) Discriminating

2. Which of the following is a common stereotype about the elderly?
   (A) Elderly people have sharp memories.
   (B) Elderly people are sexually active.
   (C) Elderly people are less intelligent than younger people.
   (D) Elderly people are very independent.

3. Most older people
   (A) Do not like to leave home
   (B) Are active and have many interests
   (C) Cannot manage their money
   (D) Are ill and dependent

12. Discuss developmental disabilities

True or False

1. ____ Developmental disabilities are present at birth or emerge during childhood.

2. ____ Developmental disabilities cause difficulty with language, learning, and self-care.

3. ____ The most common developmental disability is autism spectrum disorder.

Name: _____

4. ____ People who have developmental disabilities prefer to be treated like children.

6

Infection Prevention

1. Review the key terms in Learning Objective 1 before completing the workbook exercises

2. Define *infection prevention* and discuss types of infections

Matching
Use each letter only once.

1. ____ Communicable disease

2. ____ Cross-infection

3. ____ Healthcare-associated infection (HAI)

4. ____ Infection prevention

5. ____ Localized infection

6. ____ Microorganism

7. ____ Pathogens

8. ____ Reinfection

9. ____ Resistance

10. ____ Systemic infection

(A) A living thing or organism that is so small that it is only visible under a microscope

(B) Infection that is in the bloodstream and is spread throughout the body

(C) The body's ability to prevent infection and disease

(D) Microorganisms that are capable of causing infection and disease

(E) Infection that is limited to a specific location in the body

(F) The physical movement or transfer of harmful bacteria from one person, object, or place to another, or from one part of the body to another

(G) An infectious disease transmissible by direct contact or by indirect contact

(H) Being infected again with the same pathogen

(I) Set of methods used to prevent and control the spread of disease

(J) An infection acquired within a healthcare setting during the delivery of medical care

3. Discuss terms related to infection prevention

True or False

1. ____ Sterilization means all microorganisms are destroyed, including those that form spores.

2. ____ Medical asepsis means that a facility is completely free from all microorganisms.

3. ____ A nursing assistant (NA) must wash his hands before leaving a dirty utility room.

4. ____ Transmission is the process of removing pathogens from an object.

5. ____ An object can be called *clean* if it has not been contaminated with pathogens.

6. ____ Spore-forming organisms, a special group of organisms that produce a protective covering that is difficult to penetrate, are killed by disinfection.

7. _____ Clean and dirty equipment, linen, and supplies are normally stored in the same utility room.

4. Describe the chain of infection

Short Answer

1. What does the chain of infection describe?

_____

_____

_____

_____

_____

_____

2. How many links in the chain of infection must be broken for infection to be prevented?

_____

3. List the six links of the chain of infection.

_____

_____

_____

_____

_____

_____

5. Explain why the elderly are at a higher risk for infection

Multiple Choice

1. One reason that older people are at a greater risk for acquiring infections is
   (A) Their bones become stronger
   (B) They are hospitalized more often
   (C) They recover more quickly from illness
   (D) Their circulation increases

2. Which of the following is a factor associated with aging that increases the risk of infection?
   (A) Thicker skin
   (B) Increased circulation
   (C) Use of catheters and other tubing
   (D) Increased mobility

6. Describe Centers for Disease Control and Prevention (CDC) and explain Standard Precautions

Fill in the Blank

1. The abbreviation for the government agency that promotes public health and safety and attempts to control and prevent disease is

   _____.

2. The two levels of precautions in the infection prevention system recommended by the CDC are Standard Precautions and

   _____

   _____.

3. Standard Precautions means treating all blood, body fluids, non-intact skin, and mucous membranes as if they were

   _____.

4. An NA cannot tell by looking at residents or even by reading their charts if they have a(n) _____ disease.

5. An NA should wear a

   _____

   and protective _____ if there is a chance of coming into contact with splashing or spraying body fluids.

6. Razor blades and other sharps should be disposed of in a _____ container for sharps.

7. An NA should never transfer

   _____ items or any kind of _____ from one room to another.

8. An NA should never place

   _____ items like bedpans on an overbed table.

9. When cleaning anything, the NA should move from the

_____ to the

_____ area.

7. Define *hand hygiene* and identify when to wash hands

True or False

1. _____ Handwashing is the single most important method to reduce the spread of infection.

2. _____ Bacteria can be removed from artificial nails with thorough handwashing.

3. _____ The use of hand lotion can prevent skin from cracking.

4. _____ A nursing assistant must wash her hands every time she removes her gloves.

5. _____ A nursing assistant must wash his hands after he blows his nose.

6. _____ A nursing assistant does not need to wash her hands before obtaining clean linen from a cart.

7. _____ When washing hands, the nursing assistant should use friction for no more than five seconds.

8. _____ Using alcohol-based hand rubs means that nursing assistants do not need to wash their hands with soap and water.

8. Discuss the use of personal protective equipment (PPE) in facilities

Multiple Choice

1. Which of the following is the main factor that determines what type of personal protective equipment (PPE) must be worn for a specific task?
   (A) The type of exposure that may be encountered
   (B) The resident's preference on what type of PPE should be worn
   (C) Whether or not specific kinds of PPE are big enough to fit the nursing assistant
   (D) How comfortable the resident's family is with the choice of PPE

2. What is the step that the nursing assistant should take directly after removing and discarding PPE?
   (A) Gathering clean PPE for the next task
   (B) Restocking glove boxes
   (C) Performing hand hygiene
   (D) Documenting resident care

3. If a gown becomes wet during care, what should the nursing assistant do?
   (A) Dry it with clean paper towels
   (B) Remove the gown and shake it gently until it air dries
   (C) Spot clean the wet areas with a bleach solution
   (D) Discard it and don a new gown

4. Immediately after giving care, what should the nursing assistant do with his gloves?
   (A) He should wash his gloves.
   (B) He should don a second pair of gloves over the first pair.
   (C) He should remove the gloves and wash his hands.
   (D) He should check the gloves for holes and if they are not torn, he should keep them on for use with the next resident.

5. Which of the following should be worn when it is likely that blood or body fluids may be splashed into the eyes?
   (A) Goggles
   (B) Hat
   (C) Eyeglasses
   (D) Sunglasses

Name: _____

Short Answer

Make a check mark (✓) next to the tasks that require a nursing assistant to wear gloves.

1. ____ Contact with body fluids

2. ____ Hanging laundry

3. ____ When the NA may touch blood

4. ____ Brushing a resident's hair

5. ____ Assisting with perineal care

6. ____ Giving a massage to a resident with acne on his back

7. ____ Hugging a resident

8. ____ Shaving a resident

9. List guidelines for handling linen and equipment

Crossword Puzzle

Across

4. Type of container in which sharps should be disposed

5. Linen should be rolled so that the dirtiest area is here

6. Nursing assistants should not do this to dirty linen or clothes

Down

1. Another word for single-use equipment

2. Must be worn when handling soiled linen

3. Abbreviation for federal government agency that sets guidelines for the storage and disposal of linens and equipment

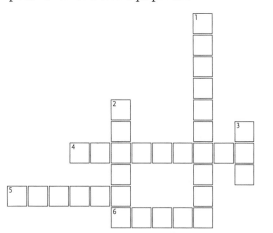

10. Explain how to handle spills

Short Answer

1. Why are spills in a healthcare facility dangerous?

_____

_____

_____

_____

2. When something is spilled, what is the first step that a nursing assistant should take?

_____

_____

_____

_____

_____

3. If a nursing assistant spills a substance on her body, what should she do?

_____

_____

_____

_____

_____

11. Discuss Transmission-Based Precautions

Short Answer

Write the first letter of the correct type of precaution ("A" for Airborne, "D" for Droplet, or "C" for Contact) for each of the following.

1. ____ *Clostridium difficile* (*C. diff*) is an example of an infection requiring these type of precautions.

2. ____ Transmission of a microorganism can occur with direct contact, for example, a nursing assistant bathing a resident.

3. ____ These precautions reduce the risk of spreading tuberculosis.

4. ____ Microorganisms can be spread by talking, singing, sneezing, laughing, or coughing.

5. ____ Diseases can be transmitted through the air.

6. ____ Infection can be spread by touching contaminated personal items.

12. Describe care of the resident in an isolation unit

Short Answer

1. If it is allowed, why is it important for a nursing assistant to spend as much time as possible with a resident who is in isolation?

_____

_____

_____

_____

_____

_____

2. Which type of supplies are best for residents in isolation?

_____

_____

_____

_____

3. What are items that may be needed when setting up an isolation cart?

_____

_____

_____

_____

_____

_____

13. Explain OSHA's Bloodborne Pathogen Standard

Word Search

1. _____ is the abbreviation of the government agency that regulates the safety of workers in the United States.

2. The _____

_____ Standard is the law that requires healthcare facilities to protect employees from blood-borne health hazards.

3. A(n) _____

_____ is when an employee is exposed to blood or other potentially infectious material.

4. A(n) _____

_____ plan outlines specific work practices to prevent exposure to infectious material and identifies step-by-step procedures to follow when exposures do occur.

5. In the healthcare setting, contact with

_____or

_____ is the most common way to be infected with a bloodborne disease.

6. The employer is responsible for providing a free _____ vaccine to all employees after hire.

14. Discuss two important bloodborne diseases

Multiple Choice

1. How does the human immunodeficiency virus (HIV) cause the body to be unable to fight infection?
   (A) It causes cirrhosis.
   (B) It causes liver cancer.
   (C) It weakens the immune system.
   (D) It poisons the blood.

2. What is one way that HIV is spread?
   (A) By coughing or sneezing
   (B) By using infected needles
   (C) By hugging
   (D) Through handshakes

3. Hepatitis ____ and ____ are bloodborne diseases that can cause death.
   (A) A and B
   (B) B and C
   (C) C and E
   (D) A and C

4. Which of the following statements is true of hepatitis B?
   (A) Hepatitis B is commonly spread by the fecal-oral route.
   (B) There is no vaccine for hepatitis B.
   (C) Hepatitis B can be spread by contact with infected needles.
   (D) Hepatitis B can be spread through contaminated water.

15. Discuss MRSA, VRE, and C. *Difficile*, and CRE

True or False

1. ____ Multidrug-resistant organisms (MDROs) are not a serious problem in healthcare facilities.

2. ____ Methicillin-resistant *Staphylococcus aureus* (MRSA) is mostly spread by direct physical contact with infected people.

3. ____ Proper hand hygiene can help prevent the spread of vancomycin-resistant *enterococcus* (VRE).

4. ____ The bacteria *enterococci* often causes problems in healthy people.

5. ____ Both hand rubs and washing hands with soap and water are considered equally effective when dealing with *C. difficile*.

6. ____ The overuse of antibiotics may alter the normal intestinal flora and increase the risk of developing *C. difficile* diarrhea.

7. ____ There is no test that can diagnose *C. difficile*.

8. ____ Carbapenem-resistant *Enterobacteriaceae* (CRE) is most often spread through direct contact with an infected person.

9. ____ To help protect against the spread of influenza (the flu), a person should maintain a distance of at least two feet from an infected person.

10. ____ Norovirus is not a type of contagious virus.

7

Safety and Body Mechanics

1. Review the key terms in Learning Objective 1 before completing the workbook exercises

2. List common accidents in facilities and ways to prevent them

True or False

1. _____ An important way that nursing assistants (NAs) can help prevent falls is to respond to call lights promptly.

2. _____ Wearing long clothing and going without shoes are helpful in preventing falls.

3. _____ A nursing assistant must identify each resident before providing care or serving food.

4. _____ Disoriented or confused residents should not be identified before serving food since they do not understand who they are.

5. _____ Burns can cause a rapid deterioration in a resident's condition.

6. _____ In order to help prevent burns, the water temperature should be 130°F when giving a bath.

7. _____ Liquids can cause burns.

8. _____ A disoriented resident may eat hair care products or flowers.

9. _____ To aid in choking prevention, residents should eat quickly.

10. _____ Sitting up straight while eating helps prevent choking.

11. _____ Large pieces of food are less likely to cause choking.

12. _____ Protecting arms and legs while moving residents helps prevent injury.

13. _____ If an NA needs help lifting a resident but nobody is around, she should lift the resident anyway.

14. _____ If no eye wash station is available after an eye splash, the NA should rinse his eye immediately with water at a sink.

3. Explain the Safety Data Sheet (SDS)

Short Answer

1. List five examples of information that is found on a Safety Data Sheet (SDS).

_____

_____

_____

_____

_____

_____

_____

2. What are two things that a nursing assistant must know about the SDS?

_____

_____

_____

_____

10. Identify safety guidelines for intravenous (IV) lines

Fill in the Blank

1. A resident with an IV is receiving
   _____,
   nutrition, or _____
   through a vein.

2. A nursing assistant should always wear
   _____
   if she has to touch the IV area.

3. The arm that has an IV line should not be
   used to measure _____
   _____.

4. The IV tubing should not be
   _____.

5. The NA should not disconnect the IV line
   from the _____ or
   turn off the
   _____.

6. If the needle or
   _____ has fallen
   out or moves out of the vein, the NA should
   report to the nurse.

7. An _____
   is the administration of fluids into sur-
   rounding tissue.

8. The NA should report to the nurse if the
   resident complains of
   _____
   or has difficulty _____.

11. Discuss fire safety and explain the RACE and PASS acronyms

Multiple Choice

1. What are the three things needed for a fire
   to occur?
   (A) Heat, cold, matches
   (B) Heat, fuel, oxygen
   (C) Heat, nitrogen, oxygen
   (D) Heat, electrical current, fuel

2. PASS is an acronym used to explain how
   to operate a fire extinguisher. The letters
   stand for
   (A) Pull the pin, Aim at the base of the fire,
   Squeeze the handle, Sweep back and
   forth at the base
   (B) Push the handle, Aim at the base of the
   fire, Spray the water, Sweep back and
   forth at the base
   (C) Push the extinguisher, Aim at the fire,
   Squeeze the handle, Spray in a circle
   (D) Pull the pin, Access the lock, Squeeze
   the handle, Spray from top of the fire
   down

3. If clothing catches fire, it is best for the per-
   son to
   (A) Jump up and down to fan the flames
   (B) Stay still and drop to the ground
   (C) Start running
   (D) Find a buddy to exit the area together

12. List general safety steps for working in a healthcare facility

True or False

1. _____ Living or working in a facility means
   a person is safe from all crime.

2. _____ Very few people go in and out of a
   facility during the day.

3. _____ It is best for a nursing assistant to
   watch for suspicious behavior and
   report it immediately.

4. _____ It is a smart idea for a nursing assistant to take valuables to work so that
   he can keep an eye on them.

5. _____ A nursing assistant should not leave
   a resident alone with a visitor or staff
   member who makes her uneasy.

6. _____ To promote safety, an NA should
   share her personal information with
   anyone who asks.

8

Emergency Care, First Aid, and Disasters

1. Review the key terms in Learning Objective 1 before completing the workbook exercises

2. Demonstrate how to respond to medical emergencies

Short Answer

1. When a nursing assistant is assessing an emergency situation, what should he do?

_____

_____

_____

_____

_____

2. When a nursing assistant is assessing a victim in a medical emergency, what should he do?

_____

_____

_____

_____

_____

_____

_____

_____

_____

_____

_____

_____

_____

_____

3. Demonstrate knowledge of first aid procedures

Crossword Puzzle

Across

2. Medical term for vomiting

4. Sudden stopping/cessation of the heartbeat

5. Medical term for fainting or temporary loss of consciousness

Down

1. Stopping/cessation of breathing

3. Way to help someone who is choking by placing both hands around a person's waist and pulling inward and upward

4. Abbreviation for medical procedures used when a person's heart and lungs have stopped working

Name: _____

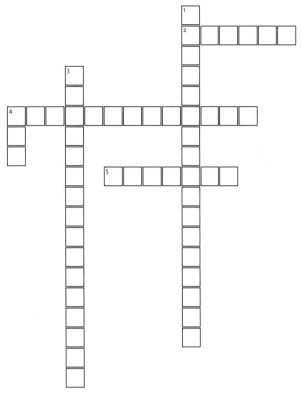

True or False

1. ____ Normally when a person is choking, she lies face down on the ground.

2. ____ The nursing assistant should leave a choking victim alone in order to find someone to help her.

3. ____ Before giving abdominal thrusts, the nursing assistant should ask the victim if he is choking.

4. ____ A person in shock should sit upright until symptoms improve.

5. ____ After notifying the nurse, the first step a nursing assistant should take when trying to control bleeding is to put on gloves.

6. ____ When blood seeps through a pad that is being used to control bleeding, it should be removed and replaced with a clean pad.

7. ____ Applying butter to a serious burn will help reduce the chance of infection.

8. ____ If a person appears likely to faint and is sitting down, the nursing assistant should have her bend forward and put her head between her knees.

9. ____ The medical term for fainting is *epistaxis*.

10. ____ When a person has vomited, it is important to check vomitus for blood or medication.

11. ____ Men are more likely than women to deny that they are having a heart attack.

12. ____ If a nursing assistant suspects a person is having a heart attack, she should give him water right away.

13. ____ The medical term for a heart attack is *transient ischemic attack (TIA)*.

14. ____ Insulin reaction results from too much insulin or too little food.

15. ____ Diabetic ketoacidosis may be caused by undiagnosed diabetes.

16. ____ If a resident is having a seizure, the nursing assistant should put his fingers inside the resident's mouth to clear any food.

17. ____ The response time to a suspected stroke is important, as early treatment can reduce severity of the stroke.

18. ____ Slurring of words and facial droop are two important signs to report that may signal a stroke is beginning.

Matching
For each sign or symptom or response described below, write the letter of the medical emergency it applies to. Use each letter only once.

1. ____ Signs of this include pale or cyanotic skin, staring, increased pulse and respiration rates, low blood pressure, and extreme thirst.

2. ____ The NA should hold a thick sterile pad directly against the wound.

3. ____ Signs of this include severe pain in the chest, anxiety, and heartburn or indigestion.

4. ____ Performing abdominal thrusts may help with this emergency.

5. ____ The NA should apply firm pressure on both sides of the nose, up near the bridge, if this occurs.

6. ____ Ointment, salve, or grease should not be used on this.

7. ____ If a person is sitting, the NA can have her bend forward and place her head between her knees if she is able.

8. ____ Signs of this include use of inappropriate words, loss of bowel and bladder control, and arm numbness.

9. ____ When this occurs, the NA should not try to stop it or hold the person down.

10. ____ Sweet or fruity breath is a symptom.

11. ____ If this occurs, it is a good idea to give the person a glass of fruit juice or milk immediately.

12. ____ Providing oral care after this happens is helpful.

13. ____ Signs of this include vomiting and heavy, difficult breathing.

(A) Bleeding

(B) Burn

(C) Choking

(D) Diabetic ketoacidosis

(E) Fainting (syncope)

(F) Insulin reaction (hypoglycemia)

(G) Myocardial infarction

(H) Nosebleed (epistaxis)

(I) Poisoning

(J) Seizure

(K) Shock

(L) Stroke

(M) Vomiting (emesis)

4. Explain the nursing assistant's role on a code team

Fill in the Blank

1. Facilities use codes to inform staff of _____ without alarming residents and visitors.

2. *Code Red* usually means _____, and *Code Blue* usually means _____.

3. The _____ is the team chosen for a shift to respond in case of a resident emergency.

4. Staff on the code team may be asked to get a special _____ or other emergency equipment.

5. Nursing assistants may be asked to perform _____ during CPR.

5. Describe guidelines for responding to disasters

Short Answer

1. What kinds of disasters are most likely to occur in your area?

2. Describe the way nursing assistants should respond to disasters.

Name: _____

_____
_____
_____
_____
_____
_____
_____
_____
_____
_____
_____
_____
_____
_____

2. List five reasons why moving into a care facility is a big emotional adjustment for new residents.

_____
_____
_____
_____
_____
_____
_____
_____
_____

4. Describe the nursing assistant's role in the admission process

True or False

1. ____ In order to keep a new resident occupied, the nursing assistant should let him figure out how to use the bed controls and the call light.

2. ____ Family and friends are a helpful source of information for a resident's personal preferences, history, and routines.

3. ____ A new resident's admission pack may include soap, a bedpan, and a water pitcher and cup.

4. ____ It is better for the nursing assistant to wait until the resident has already arrived to start preparing her room.

5. ____ The resident should not feel as if he is an inconvenience; he should feel welcome and wanted.

6. ____ It is important for the nursing assistant to introduce new residents to other residents and staff members.

7. ____ Baseline measurements are taken approximately six months after a resident is admitted to a care facility.

8. ____ A change in a resident's weight does not need to be reported as long as the gain or loss is within five pounds.

9. ____ Residents who cannot get out of bed cannot have their height or weight measured.

10. ____ When measuring height, the nursing assistant should remember that there are eight inches in a foot.

5. Explain the nursing assistant's role during an in-house transfer of a resident

Fill in the Blank

1. Residents may need to be transferred to a unit that offers more

    _____ care.

2. _____ is always hard. This may be especially true if the resident is _____ or his condition has

    _____.

3. Nursing assistants should try to make the transfer as _____ as possible for residents.

4. The nursing assistant should
_____ the resident's personal items carefully to avoid damaging or losing them.

5. After the resident is in her new room, the nursing assistant should
_____ her to everyone.

6. When leaving the resident's room, the nursing assistant should report to the

_____

in charge of the resident.

6. Explain the nursing assistant's role in the discharge of a resident

Multiple Choice

1. When does a resident's discharge from the facility become official?
   (A) After the doctor writes the discharge order that releases the resident to leave the facility
   (B) After the resident is informed of the discharge
   (C) After the resident leaves the facility
   (D) When the nurse gives the resident instructions to be followed after discharge

2. Which of the following is the nursing assistant's responsibility during discharge?
   (A) Collecting and packing the resident's belongings
   (B) Giving the resident any special dietary instructions
   (C) Writing the discharge order
   (D) Reviewing medications that the resident needs to take

3. A nursing assistant is responsible for the resident until
   (A) The discharge order has been written by the doctor
   (B) The resident's items are packed, and the inventory list has been checked
   (C) The resident is outside the facility
   (D) The resident is safely in the vehicle with the doors closed

7. Describe the nursing assistant's role during physical exams

Multiple Choice

1. What are the nursing assistant's duties during residents' physical exams?
   (A) Performing the exams
   (B) Giving injections
   (C) Diagnosing illness or disease
   (D) Gathering equipment for the doctor or nurse

2. In which position is the resident placed for examination of the breasts, chest, abdomen, and perineal area?
   (A) Dorsal recumbent position
   (B) Lithotomy position
   (C) Knee-chest position
   (D) Trendelenburg position

3. Which of the following pieces of equipment is used to measure blood pressure?
   (A) Reflex hammer
   (B) Thermometer
   (C) Sphygmomanometer
   (D) Otoscope

4. In which position is the resident in stirrups in order to examine the vagina?
   (A) Sims' position
   (B) Lithotomy position
   (C) Knee-chest position
   (D) Prone position

5. Which position is used to examine the rectum or the vagina?
   (A) Lateral position
   (B) Lithotomy position
   (C) Knee-chest position
   (D) Prone position

Name: _____

10

Bedmaking and Unit Care

1. Review the key terms in Learning Objective 1 before completing the workbook exercises

2. Discuss the importance of sleep

Fill in the Blank

1. _____ is a natural period of rest for the mind and body during which _____ is restored.

2. Sleep is needed to replace old _____ with new ones and provide new energy to _____.

3. _____ are natural rhythms and cycles related to body functions.

4. The _____ is the 24-hour day-night cycle.

3. Describe types of sleep disorders

Matching
Use each letter only once.

1. ____ Bruxism

2. ____ Insomnia

3. ____ Parasomnias

4. ____ REM behavior disorder

5. ____ Sleep apnea

6. ____ Sleeptalking

7. ____ Somnambulism

(A) Talking during sleep

(B) Grinding and clenching the teeth

(C) Sleepwalking

(D) Inability to fall asleep or to remain asleep

(E) Sleep disorders

(F) Talking, often along with violent movements, during REM sleep

(G) Disruption of breathing while sleeping

4. Identify factors affecting sleep

Scenario
Read the following scenario and answer the questions that follow.

New resident Anne Ross has been having trouble sleeping. She generally has dinner, dessert, and coffee around 8:30 p.m. every day. Her husband recently died in the home they shared together for 24 years. After his death, she started a new medication to help with her depression. Her roommate, Riva, likes to sleep with the light on because she frequently has to use the bathroom. Sometimes Riva is unable to make it to the bathroom in time and has to call a nursing assistant for help. The nursing assistant will change the sheets and help Riva clean herself as quickly as possible.

1. List five factors that could be affecting Anne's ability to sleep.

_____

_____

_____

_____

Name: _____

Bedmaking and Unit Care